D1722082

THE

KIDNEY AND FATTY

LIVER CURE

Revitalize Your Body, Boost Your Energy, and Transform Your Health with the Ultimate Guide to Reversing Kidney Disease and Fatty Liver

Dr. Cynthia R. Norton

Copyright © 2023, Dr. Cynthia R. Norton.

Table of Contents

Introduction

Linda had been struggling with her health for years. Her doctor had diagnosed her with both kidney and liver disease, and she had tried everything to alleviate her symptoms. She had been on various medications, tried different diets, and even considered surgery. But nothing seemed to work.

One day, while browsing through a bookstore, Linda stumbled upon a book called "The Kidney and Fatty Liver Cure." Intrigued, she decided to purchase it and give it a read.

As she delved into the book, Linda learned about the importance of a healthy diet, regular exercise, and various natural remedies that could help improve her condition. She was amazed at how much she didn't know about her health and how simple changes to her lifestyle could make a significant difference.

Linda became dedicated to following the book's advice, making changes to her diet, and incorporating exercise into her daily routine. She also started taking natural supplements recommended in the book.

To her delight, Linda began to notice a significant improvement in her health. Her energy levels increased, and she was no longer experiencing the debilitating symptoms that had plagued her for so long. When she went back to her doctor for a check-up, he was surprised at how much her condition had improved.

Linda couldn't believe how much of a difference the book had made in her life. She felt like she had been given a second chance, and she was grateful for the knowledge and guidance she had received from the book. She made a promise to herself to continue living a healthy lifestyle, and she knew that she had the book to thank for her renewed health and vitality.

The Force of the Kidney and Fatty Liver Cure. The Kidney and Fatty Liver Cure is a characteristic cure that assists with supporting the body's innate capacity to purge and detoxify the kidneys and liver. This cure consists of normal fixings that are accepted to help the body's regular purifying interaction. The fixings are explicitly decided to assist with advancing the end of poisons, while likewise offering regular help to the kidneys and liver in their capability. This cure has been utilized by well-being experts for a really long time to assist with working on by and large well-being and health. It is an incredible approach to normally enhance your eating regimen and furnish your body with the help it requires to stay sound and work at its ideal.

The fixings in the Kidney and Fatty Liver Cure are painstakingly decided to assist with supporting the body's regular detoxification and purging cycle. These fixings incorporate spices, nutrients, minerals, and other regular substances that help the body's normal capabilities. These fixings cooperate to assist the body with flushing out poisons and different pollutants, while additionally offering help to the kidneys and liver. This cure is protected and successful and can be taken every day to offer continuous help for the body's normal purifying and detoxification process.

The Kidney and Fatty Liver Cure is an incredible method for supporting your body's inherent capacity to purge and detoxify itself. This cure consists of normal fixings that are decided to assist with advancing the disposal of poisons, while additionally offering regular help to the kidneys and greasy liver in their capability. This cure is protected, extremely compelling, and can be taken day to day to offer continuous help for the body's regular purging and detoxification process.

By taking the Kidney and Fatty Liver Cure, you can assist with supporting your body's innate capacity to purge and detoxify itself. This regular cure is an extraordinary approach to normally enhance your eating routine and furnish your body with the help it requires to stay sound and work at its ideal.

Much obliged to you for carving out the opportunity to find out about the Kidney and Fatty Liver Cure. We trust this presentation has been useful in providing you with a superior comprehension of this normal cure and how it can assist with supporting your body's regular purging and detoxification process.

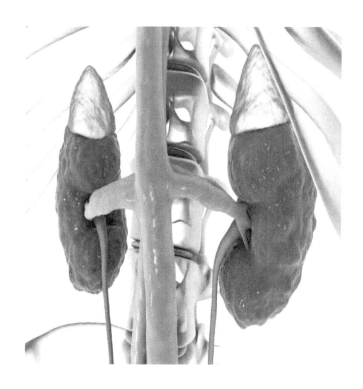

Chapter 1: Understanding the Basics of the Kidney and Fatty Liver Cure

Understanding the Basics of the Kidney:

The kidney is a vital organ in the human body responsible for filtering waste and excess fluids from the blood. It also helps to regulate blood pressure, maintain electrolyte balance, and produce hormones that stimulate red blood cell production and control calcium metabolism.

The kidney is made up of tiny structures called nephrons, which are responsible for filtering the blood. Each nephron contains a glomerulus, which is a small network of capillaries that filters the blood, and a tubule, which collects the filtered fluid and returns it to the bloodstream.

If the kidneys are not functioning properly, waste products and excess fluids can build up in the body, leading to various health problems. Chronic kidney disease (CKD) is a condition in which the kidneys gradually lose their ability to function over time. Common causes of CKD include high blood pressure, diabetes, and kidney infections.

Treatment for CKD may involve medications, lifestyle changes (such as diet and exercise), and in severe cases, dialysis or a kidney transplant.

Understanding Fatty Liver Cure:

Fatty liver disease is a condition in which excess fat builds up in the liver. It can be caused by various factors, including obesity, high cholesterol, and excessive alcohol consumption. If left untreated, fatty liver disease can progress to more serious conditions such as liver cirrhosis and liver cancer.

The primary treatment for fatty liver disease is lifestyle changes. This includes losing weight, following a healthy diet, and getting regular exercise. In addition, avoiding alcohol and managing any underlying medical conditions such as diabetes or high cholesterol can also help improve the condition.

Medications may also be used to treat fatty liver disease. These may include drugs that help to lower cholesterol, reduce inflammation, and improve insulin resistance.

In some cases, fatty liver disease may require more invasive treatment. For example, if the liver is severely damaged, a liver transplant may be necessary.

The kidney and the liver are two important organs in the human body that play crucial roles in maintaining overall health. Understanding the basics of how these organs function, as well as the causes and treatments for common conditions such as chronic kidney disease and fatty liver disease, can help individuals take steps to maintain their health and prevent complications. If you are experiencing symptoms related to these organs, it is important to speak with a healthcare provider to determine the best course of treatment.

1. Eat a sound eating routine: A reasonable eating regimen of new foods grown from the ground, lean proteins, entire grains, and low-fat dairy items is fundamental for keeping up with kidney and liver well-being.

2. Work out consistently: Normal activity assists with lessening the gamble of creating persistent kidney and liver illnesses.

3.   Decrease   your   liquor consumption: Drinking an excessive amount of liquor can prompt serious liver harm and kidney issues.

4. Abstain from smoking: Smoking expands the gamble of creating kidney and liver issues.

5. Screen your prescriptions: A few drugs can be destructive to the kidneys or liver. Make certain to inform your PCP regarding all drugs you are taking.

6. Get ordinary check-ups: Getting normal check-ups from your primary care physician can assist with distinguishing any potential issues almost immediately and assist with keeping them from turning out to be more serious.

7. Keep a sound weight: Being overweight builds the gamble of creating kidney and liver issues.

8. Drink a lot of water: Remaining very much hydrated assists with flushing out poisons from the body, which can assist with safeguarding the kidneys and liver.

Anatomy and Physiology of the Kidney and Liver

The kidney and liver are two of the main organs in the human body. They are answerable for the vast majority of essential capabilities, and when they don't work as expected, they can have significant results.

The life systems of the kidney incorporate the renal cortex, which is the external layer of the organ and contains the glomeruli, which are answerable for sifting side effects from the blood. The renal medulla is the internal layer of the kidney, and it contains the renal tubules, which reabsorb significant substances from the separated liquid. The renal pelvis is a pipe-like construction that gathers the sifted liquid and leads it to the ureter.

The life systems of the liver incorporate the curves, which are the four divisions of the organ. The curves are isolated into left and right parts, and they contain the hepatic lobules, which are useful units of the liver. The lobules are made out of hepatocytes, which are the cells that produce bile, a substance that assists the body with processing fats.

The physiology of the kidney includes the filtration of the blood, reabsorption of specific substances, and the creation of pee. The glomeruli channel the blood, and the renal tubules reabsorb significant substances like glucose, amino acids, and electrolytes. The renal pelvis gathers the separated liquid and leads it to the ureter, which conveys the pee to the bladder.

The physiology of the liver includes the development of bile, which assists the body with processing fats, the digestion of proteins, lipids, and starches, and the stockpiling of glycogen, which is a type of energy that the body can get to when required. The liver additionally delivers and secretes a few chemicals and assists with freeing the collection of poisons.

Taking everything into account, the life systems and physiology of the kidney and liver are mind-boggling and interrelated. The two organs are fundamental for the appropriate working of the body and can be unfavorably impacted by different infections and conditions. A sound way of life and normal exams with your PCP can assist with keeping your organs working appropriately.

Common Symptoms of Kidney Disease include:

1. Diminished pee yield: Kidney sickness can cause a decline in how much pee is delivered. This can be because of a reduction in the development of the chemical that manages how much water and salt are in the body, or it very well may be brought about by a lessening in the number of practical nephrons in the kidneys.

2. Liquid maintenance: Liquid maintenance, or edema, can be a side effect of kidney sickness. This happens when the kidneys can't channel waste and overabundance of liquid from the blood, making the body hold additional liquid which can prompt an expansion in the face, hands, lower legs, and feet.

3. Expanding: Enlarging can happen because of the development of byproducts in the body, or because of liquid maintenance. It is much of the time found in the hands, feet, lower legs, and face.

4. Exhaustion: Weariness can be a side effect of various illnesses, including kidney sickness. This happens when the body experiences issues sifting waste and poisons through the body, prompting sensations of outrageous sluggishness and depletion.

5. Tingling: Tingling is in many cases a side effect of kidney illness. This can happen because of the collection of side effects in the skin, or because of dryness made by the failure of the kidneys appropriately channel electrolytes.

6. Sickness and regurgitation: Queasiness and retching can happen because of the development of side effects in the body, or because of prescriptions used to treat kidney illness.

7. Windedness: Windedness can be a side effect of kidney sickness. This happens when the body experiences issues sifting oxygen from the blood, prompting trouble relaxing.

8. Loss of hunger: Loss of craving can be a side effect of kidney sickness. This happens when the body experiences issues separating side effects from the blood, prompting decreased hunger.

9. Muscle cramps: Muscle issues can be a side effect of kidney sickness. This happens when the body experiences issues sifting electrolytes from the blood, prompting muscle cramps.

10. Hypertension: Hypertension can be a side effect of kidney illness. This happens when the kidneys can't sift through waste and electrolytes from the blood, prompting expanded tension in the veins.

Common Symptoms Of Fatty Liver Disease

1. Exhaustion: Weariness is a typical side effect of liver infection, for what it's worth for the overwhelming majority of different circumstances.

2. Jaundice: This is the yellow staining of the skin and eyes because of the development of bilirubin in the circulatory system.

3. Stomach expanding: This can be brought about by a development of liquid in the midsection (ascites), which is many times brought about by liver sickness.

4. Queasiness and heaving: This can be a side effect of various liver illnesses, including hepatitis, cirrhosis, and liver malignant growth.

5. Dull shaded pee: This can be an indication of liver infection, as the liver is answerable for sifting through poisons and side effects from the body.

6. Light-shaded stools: This can be an indication of bile channel impediment, which can be brought about by various liver illnesses.

7. Hunger misfortune: This can be an indication of various liver illnesses, as well as different circumstances.

8. Tingling: This is in many cases brought about by the development of bile salts in the skin, which can be an indication of liver sickness.

9. Weight reduction: This can be a side effect of various liver infections, including hepatitis and cirrhosis.

10. Simple swelling or dying: This can be an indication of liver sickness, as the liver is liable for delivering the coagulating factors that assist with halting dying.

Benefits of the Kidney and Fatty Liver Cure

The Benefits Of Kidney Cure Are:

1. Worked on Cardiovascular Well-being: The kidneys help to direct pulse, and when they are working appropriately, they can assist with lessening the general hazard of stroke, coronary episodes, and other cardiovascular issues.

2. Further developed Kidney Capability: Individuals who have solid kidneys can sift through side effects and poisons from the body. This assists with forestalling kidney disappointment and other kidney-related conditions.

3. Worked on Stomach related Well-being: The kidneys help to direct electrolyte balance, which is significant for keeping up with stomach-related well-being. At the point when the kidneys are working appropriately, they can assist with diminishing side effects of blockage, gas, bulging, and queasiness.

4. Security from Contaminations: The kidneys help to sift through microscopic organisms and different poisons from the body. At the point when the kidneys are working appropriately, they can assist with safeguarding against contaminations and different ailments.

5. Diminished Hazard of Disease:
The kidneys help to direct chemicals in the body. At the point when the kidneys are working appropriately, they can assist with diminishing the gamble of particular kinds of diseases, like kidney and bladder malignant growth.

6. Worked on Resistant Framework: The kidneys help to direct the body's insusceptible framework. At the point when the kidneys are working appropriately, they can assist with diminishing the general gamble of disease and ailment.

7. Further developed Digestion:
The kidneys help to direct the body's

digestion, which is significant for keeping a solid weight. At the point when the kidneys are working appropriately, they can assist with lessening the general gamble of corpulence and other metabolic problems.

8. Worked on Mental Capability:
The kidneys help to direct the body's electrolyte balance, which is significant for keeping up with general mental well-being. At the point when the kidneys are working appropriately, they can assist with diminishing the gamble old enough related mental deterioration.

9. Diminished Hazard of Diabetes:
The kidneys help to control blood

glucose levels, which is significant for lessening the gamble of creating diabetes. At the point when the kidneys are working appropriately, they can assist with diminishing generally speaking gamble of this constant condition.

10. Worked on Psychological wellness: The kidneys help to manage chemicals in the body, which can affect emotional well-being. At the point when the kidneys are working appropriately, they can assist with decreasing the gamble of specific emotional well-being conditions, like sadness and nervousness.

The Benefits Of Fatty Liver Cure Are:

The liver is quite possibly the main organ in the human body, carrying out various crucial roles. It is liable for separating and separating poisons, creating bile to support absorption, putting away supplements, and delivering proteins that are fundamental for coagulating. Here is a portion of the top advantages of the liver:

1. Detoxification: The liver is a significant purging organ, fit for separating and breaking down poisons, like liquor, drugs, and ecological contaminations. Doing this will assist with shielding the body from these hurtful substances.

2. Stomach-related Help: The liver produces bile, which assists with separating fats and different parts of food during absorption. This makes it more straightforward for the body to assimilate fundamental supplements.

3. Nutrient Capacity: The liver stores significant nutrients, like A, D, E, and K, which can be utilized when required.

4. Protein Creation: The liver is answerable for delivering proteins, for example, egg whites and coagulation factors, which are fundamental for legitimate blood thickening.

5. Metabolic Guideline: The liver is engaged with various metabolic exercises, including the development of glucose, the guideline of cholesterol levels, and the change of putting away fats into energy.

Generally, the liver is an essential organ, assuming a critical part of the strength of the whole body. It is fundamental for detoxification, supporting absorption, putting away nutrients, creating proteins, and controlling digestion.

Notwithstanding its numerous medical advantages, the liver is likewise exceptionally versatile and can recover itself after harm. Subsequently, it is essential to deal with your liver and safeguard it from hurt. Eating a fair eating regimen, restricting liquor consumption, and keeping away from specific meds and poisons can assist with keeping your liver working ideally.

On the off chance that you are encountering any side effects of liver sickness, like jaundice, stomach agony, queasiness, or weakness, looking for clinical attention is significant. Early finding and treatment of liver issues can assist with lessening the gamble of serious inconveniences.

By dealing with your liver and shielding it from hurt, you can assist with guaranteeing its ideal working and partake in the many advantages it gives.

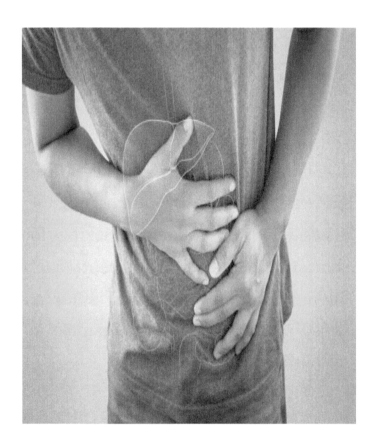

Chapter 2: Detoxification

Kidneys and the liver are essential organs that play a vital role in the body's detoxification process. The kidneys filter waste and toxins from the blood, while the liver metabolizes and removes toxins from the body. However, certain lifestyle factors, such as a high-fat diet, excessive alcohol consumption, and sedentary behavior, can damage these organs and impair their ability to function correctly.

Fatty liver disease is a condition where there is an accumulation of fat in the liver cells, leading to inflammation and damage to the liver. This condition is prevalent in people who consume a high-fat diet, are overweight, or have type 2 diabetes. When the liver is unable to function correctly, it can affect the kidneys' ability to filter waste and toxins from the blood.

Detoxification of the kidneys and liver is crucial to maintain good health and preventing the onset of diseases such as fatty liver disease. Here are some ways to detoxify your kidneys and liver naturally:

Drink plenty of water: Water is essential for the kidneys to function correctly. It helps flush out toxins and waste from the body, promoting kidney health. Drinking at least 8-10 glasses of water a day can help keep your kidneys healthy.

Eat a healthy diet: A diet rich in fruits, vegetables, and whole grains can help detoxify the liver and kidneys. Foods that are high in antioxidants, such as blueberries, cranberries, and pomegranates, can also help protect the organs from damage.

Limit alcohol consumption: Alcohol is a toxin that can damage the liver and impair its ability to function correctly. Limiting alcohol consumption or avoiding it altogether can help protect your liver and kidneys.

Exercise regularly: Regular exercise can help improve liver and kidney function by promoting blood flow to these organs. Exercise also helps reduce the risk of obesity and type 2 diabetes, which can contribute to fatty liver disease.

Get enough sleep: Getting enough sleep is crucial for the body's overall health, including the kidneys and liver. Lack of sleep can lead to inflammation, which can damage these organs over time.

The kidneys and the liver are essential organs that play a crucial role in the body's detoxification process. Maintaining good kidney and liver health is essential for overall health and well-being. By making simple lifestyle changes such as drinking plenty of water, eating a healthy diet, limiting alcohol consumption, exercising regularly, and getting enough sleep, you can help detoxify these organs and promote good health.

Detoxification is a course of taking out poisons from the body. These poisons can incorporate weighty metals like lead, mercury, cadmium, and arsenic, as well as synthetics, like pesticides and herbicides. The body has normal detoxification processes that assist with eliminating poisons, yet these cycles can be overpowered when an excessive number of poisons are available. Detoxification is utilized to assist with purifying the body of these poisons, permitting it to work all the more proficiently.

Detoxification should be possible in various ways, including dietary changes, enhancements, and exceptional purging projects. Detoxification slims down ordinarily including wiping out handled food varieties, caffeine, liquor, and sugar, and eating just regular, entire food varieties like natural products, vegetables, nuts, and seeds. Other dietary changes might incorporate expanding water admission and eating more plant-based proteins like beans, vegetables, and tempeh.

Supplements are likewise frequently utilized during detoxification to assist with supporting the body's normal detoxification processes. These can incorporate nutrients and minerals, natural cures, and probiotics.

Purifying projects can likewise be utilized to assist with detoxifying the body. These projects might include fasting, colon purging, and other detoxification techniques.

Detoxification can assist with supporting the body's regular detoxification processes and diminish the weight of poisons on the body. It can assist with further developing general medical care and might be valuable for those with ailments connected with poison over-burden.

Before beginning any detoxification program, it is critical to talk with a well-being master supplier to guarantee that it is protected and fitting.

To detoxify the framework, begin with a decent eating regimen of new food sources, homegrown teas, a lot of water, and exercise. Moreover, consider taking enhancements to help the body's regular detoxification processes and adding detoxification medicines into your daily schedule.

At last, make certain to get sufficient rest and unwind, as these are significant parts of a sound way of life.

Improved Digestive Health

1. Eat more fiber: Eating more fiber-rich food varieties, like vegetables, natural products, vegetables, nuts, and entire grains, can assist with working on your stomach-related well-being.

2. Remain hydrated: Drinking a lot of liquids assists with keeping your stomach-related framework moving along as expected.

3. Stay away from handled food varieties: Eating too many handled food sources can lead to stomach-related issues.

4. Work out routinely: Exercise assists with invigorating your stomach-related framework, which can work on its capability.

5. Decrease pressure: Stress can adversely affect your stomach-related well-being. Make a point to find the opportunity to unwind and rehearse pressure-the-board strategies.

6. Abstain from smoking and unnecessary liquor utilization: Smoking and over-the-top liquor utilization can both adversely affect your stomach-related well-being.

7. Take probiotic supplements: Probiotics are valuable microbes that assist with supporting a sound stomach-related framework. Taking a quality probiotic supplement can assist with working on stomach-related well-being.

8. Eat more modest feasts all the more much of the time: Eating more modest dinners all the more now and again over the day can assist with further developing assimilation.

9. Stay away from food sources that cause uneasiness: Assuming specific food sources cause you stomach-related distress, keeping away from them might be ideal.

10. Deal with your drugs: A few drugs can adversely affect your stomach-related well-being. Try to converse with your primary care physician about any meds you are taking.

11. Work with medical services proficiently: Working with medical services proficiently can assist with distinguishing any basic stomach-related issues and give therapy choices.

Boosted Immune System

The invulnerable framework is a perplexing organization of cells, organs, and different designs that safeguard the body from illness and disease. While our bodies normally produce the parts expected to ward off microorganisms, there are a few things we can do to support our safe framework and remain solid. The following are a couple of tips to assist you with fortifying your safe framework:

1. Eat a decent eating routine: Eating an eating routine that is wealthy in natural products, vegetables, entire grains, lean proteins, and solid fats is fundamental for helping the resistant framework. Try to incorporate a lot of cell reinforcement-rich food varieties, for example, berries, citrus natural products, and dull salad greens, which help to diminish irritation and fend off contamination.

2. Get sufficient rest: Getting sufficient rest assumes an essential part in assisting the body with warding off contamination and recuperating from sickness. Intend to get no less than 7-8 hours of rest every night to guarantee that your resistant framework is working at its ideal.

3. Work out routinely: Ordinary activity assists with decreasing pressure and lifting invulnerability by expanding dissemination and working on the body's capacity to ward off contamination. Expect to get no less than 30 minutes of moderate active work every day.

4. Oversee pressure: Stress has been connected to a debilitated insusceptible framework, so it means a lot to track down ways of overseeing and decreasing feelings of anxiety. Attempt yoga, reflection, or profound breathing activities to help you unwind and remain mentally collected.

5. Take supplements: Taking a day-to-day multivitamin or other safe helping enhancements can assist with supporting your insusceptible framework and keep it working ideally. Search for supplements that contain nutrients C, D, zinc, and selenium, which are fundamental for keeping a sound insusceptible framework.

6. Abstain from smoking and exorbitant liquor: Smoking and extreme liquor utilization can debilitate the invulnerable framework, making it harder for the body to fend off contamination and infection. On the off chance that you are a smoker, consider stopping or decreasing the sum you smoke, and breaking point how much liquor you consume.

7. Clean up: Cleaning up routinely is one of the most outstanding ways of safeguarding yourself from microbes and microscopic organisms. Utilize warm water and cleanser and scour your hands for something like 20 seconds to eliminate soil and microorganisms.

By following these tips, you can assist with supporting your invulnerable framework and diminish your gamble of disease. Keep in mind, a sound way of life is the most effective way to help your safe framework and keep it working ideally.

Assuming that you have any basic ailments, it means quite a bit to converse with your PCP before rolling out any improvements to your eating regimen or way of life.

Improved Energy Levels

Further developing your energy levels can be a test, particularly while you're feeling drained and drowsy. Luckily, there are numerous straightforward things you can do to build your energy levels, assist you with feeling more ready, and benefit from your day. Here are a few hints on the best way to further develop your energy levels:

1. Get satisfactory rest. Rest is fundamental for your body to re-energize and reestablish itself, so ensure you get enough. Go for long periods of rest every night to feel more invigorated during the day.

2. Work out consistently. Practice is one of the most amazing ways of supporting your energy levels. Besides the fact that it assists with delivering endorphins, it likewise expands your pulse, which can give you a jolt of energy. Plan to do something like 30 minutes of activity each day.

3. Eat a reasonable eating regimen. Eating a reasonable eating regimen is fundamental for keeping your energy steps up. Center around eating food sources that are high in protein, complex carbs, and solid fats. Eating more modest dinners over the day can assist with keeping your energy levels consistent.

4. Drink a lot of water. Remaining hydrated is significant for keeping your energy steps up. Expect to hydrate every day.

5. Lessen pressure. Stress can tremendously affect your energy levels, so it means quite a bit to track down ways of diminishing pressure in your life. Attempt yoga, reflection, or other pressure-lessening exercises to assist you with feeling more empowered.

6. Limit caffeine and liquor. Caffeine and liquor can give you a fast jolt of energy, however, this is trailed by an accident. Limit your admission of these

substances to keep your energy levels consistent over the day.

7. Enjoy reprieves. Enjoying reprieves over the day can assist with giving your body and psyche a rest. Attempt to require a couple of moments consistently to unwind and re-energize.

8. Get outside. Investing time in nature can assist with supporting your energy levels. Go for a stroll in the recreation area or go for a climb to get some outside air and absorb some daylight.

These are only a couple of tips on the most proficient method to further develop your energy levels. Make sure to pay attention to your body and give it the rest it needs. With a couple of straightforward changes, you can have more energy and capitalize on every day.

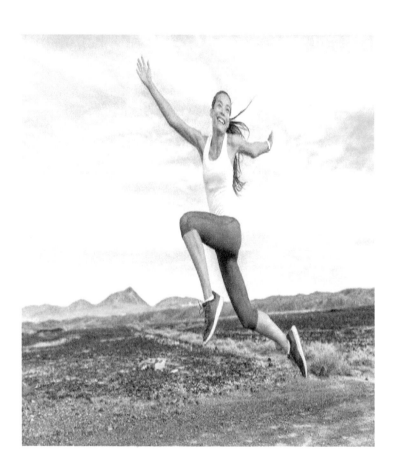

Chapter 3: How to Prepare for the Kidney and Fatty Liver Cure

Kidney and fatty liver well-being is a significant piece of general well-being and prosperity, and it's vital to deal with these organs to guarantee they stay sound. On the off chance that you're thinking about a kidney and liver purification, or fix, there are a few significant advances you ought to take to guarantee the most ideal outcomes. This is the very thing that you want to be aware of planning for a kidney and fatty liver cure.

1. Get an Examination

Before starting any sort of purge, it's critical to get an intensive actual assessment from your PCP to ensure that your organs are sound. This will permit your primary care physician to figure out what sort of scrub might work out for you and to distinguish any likely dangers.

2. Quit Taking Drugs

Certain drugs can obstruct the viability of a purge, so it's essential to converse with your PCP about any prescriptions you might be taking before starting the purification. Contingent upon the sort of purification you're doing, you might have to stop specific drugs for a specific timeframe.

3. Eat a Spotless Eating routine

Eating a spotless eating routine is crucial for the progress of any scrub. This implies staying away from handled food varieties, sugar, and refined carbs. All things considered, centers around eating entire, natural food sources like new products of the soil, lean proteins, and complex sugars.

4. Hydrate

Drinking a lot of water is critical to flushing poisons out of your body and cleaning your organs. Plan to drink no less than eight glasses of water a day, and increment your admission if you're feeling parched.

5. Take Natural Enhancements

Natural enhancements can be an extraordinary method for supporting your purge and guaranteeing the best outcomes. Search for supplements that are explicitly intended to help kidney and liver well-being, for example, milk thorn, dandelion root, and turmeric.

6. Stay away from Liquor and Caffeine

Liquor and caffeine can obstruct the viability of scrubbing, so it's ideal to keep away from these substances. On the off chance that you're accustomed to drinking liquor or espresso, wean yourself off continuously to keep away from any regrettable incidental effects.

7. Work-out Consistently

Practice is an extraordinary method for supporting your purge and keeping your organs sound. Mean to get something like 30 minutes of activity daily, or possibly three times each week.

By following these means, you can guarantee that your liver and kidney purification is protected and successful. Make sure to continuously talk with your PCP before beginning any sort of purge, and make certain to adhere to the guidelines on any enhancements you might take. With the right readiness, your purification can be an effective and compensating experience.

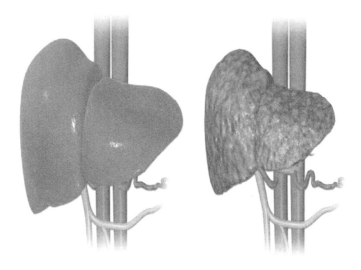

Normal Liver   Liver Cirrhosis

Chapter 4: Diet and Nutrition

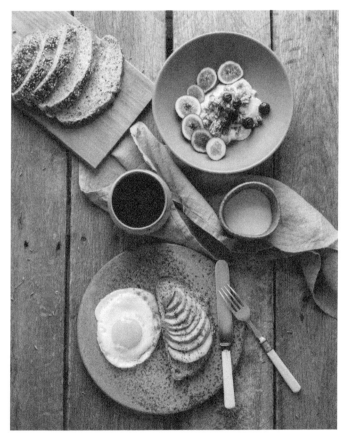

Diet and nourishment assume a significant part in the treatment of kidney and liver illnesses. A solid eating routine and way of life are significant elements in the counteraction and treatment of kidney and liver illnesses.

An eating routine to fix kidney and liver illnesses ought to incorporate food sources that are low in salt and fat, high in fiber, and loaded with fundamental nutrients and minerals. Such an eating regimen ought to incorporate a lot of new leafy foods, entire grains, vegetables, and lean proteins. Food sources that are high in sodium, like handled meats and canned soups, ought to be kept away from however much as could be expected.

Notwithstanding a sound eating regimen, it means a lot to drink a lot of liquids to appropriately assist with flushing poisons from the body and keep the kidneys and liver working. Water is the most ideal decision, however, different liquids like homegrown teas, weakened organic product squeezes, and low-sodium stocks can be valuable.

Enhancements, for example, omega-3 unsaturated fats and probiotics may likewise be helpful for kidney and liver well-being. It is essential to talk with a specialist or nutritionist before taking any enhancements to guarantee they are protected and fitting for the person.

At long last, it is vital to keep away from liquor and whatever other substances can harm the kidneys or liver. Smoking ought to likewise be stayed away from. Eating a solid, adjusted diet and taking part in standard actual work are significant stages in the treatment of kidney and liver illnesses.

By adhering to these rules, people can work on their kidney and liver well-being and lessen their gambling for intricacies.

Exercise

Exercise is one of the best ways to help improve the health of your kidneys and liver. Regular physical activity can help protect against some of the conditions that can lead to liver and kidney disease, such as obesity and diabetes. Exercise can also help improve the overall functioning of these organs, as it helps to reduce inflammation and improve circulation.

When it comes to exercising for kidney and liver health, it is important to work out in moderation. Overdoing it can be harmful to your kidneys and liver, as too much exercise can cause fatigue and dehydration. It is also important to keep your exercise routine varied, as different types of exercise can provide different benefits.

Some of the best exercises for the kidneys and liver include aerobic activities, such as walking, jogging, swimming, and biking. These exercises can help improve both your physical and mental health, as well as improve your overall circulation. Strength-training exercises, such as weight-lifting and resistance band exercises, can also be beneficial for the kidneys and liver. These exercises can help strengthen the muscles around the organs, improving their function and helping to reduce inflammation.

It is also important to stay hydrated while exercising. The kidneys and liver need plenty of fluids to help flush out toxins. Drinking plenty of water before, during, and after exercise can help keep these organs healthy.

Finally, it is important to make sure that you are getting enough rest. When you are overworked and exhausted, your kidneys and liver may not be able to function properly. Make sure to get at least 7 to 8 hours of sleep each night, as this can help ensure that your organs are functioning at their best.

By following a healthy diet, exercising regularly, and getting enough rest, you can help improve the health of your kidneys and liver. Exercise can help reduce inflammation, improve circulation, and help to strengthen the organs, allowing them to function more efficiently.

The Types Of Exercise Are:

1. Oxygen-consuming activity (for example strolling, running, swimming, cycling, and so forth.)

2. Opposition preparing (for example weightlifting, bodyweight works out, and so forth.)

3. Balance works out (for example yoga, kendo, and so forth.)

4. Extending (for example dynamic extending, static extending, and so forth.)

5. Center activities (for example boards, spans, and so forth.)

6. Stop and go aerobic exercise (HIIT)

7. Pilates

8. Aquarobics

9. Dance-based works out

10. Broadly educating (for example joining various activities).

Supplements

With regards to kidney and liver well-being, different enhancements can assist with advancing generally speaking well-being and health. The absolute most well-known supplements for kidney and liver help include:

• **Milk thorn:** Milk thorn is a spice that is known for its capacity to detoxify the liver and kidneys, as well as safeguard them from harm. It is additionally known to assist with decreasing aggravation and further developing bile creation.

• **Dandelion root:** Dandelion pull has been utilized for a long time to help liver and kidney wellbeing. It is a characteristic diuretic and can assist with flushing poisons from the body, as well as diminish irritation.

• **Turmeric:** Turmeric is a strong cell reinforcement that can assist with safeguarding the liver and kidneys. It is additionally known to decrease irritation, further develop assimilation, and lift the invulnerable framework.

• **N-Acetyl Cysteine (NAC):** NAC is an amino corrosive that is known to assist with kidney and liver capability. It can likewise assist with decreasing irritation and work on the body's capacity to detoxify itself.

• **Vitamin B Complex:** Vitamin B complex is fundamental for kidney and liver wellbeing. It assists with using proteins, carbs, and fats and can lessen aggravation.

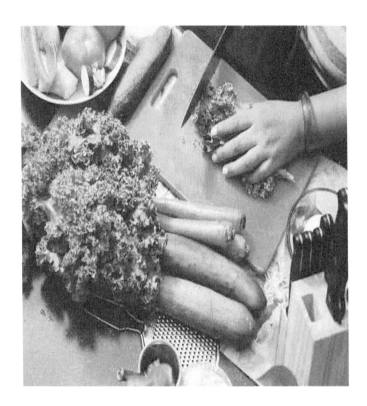

Chapter 5: The Kidney and Fatty Liver Cure Protocol

Kidney and fatty liver cure conventions for the most part include dietary alterations, way of life changes, and homegrown and healthful enhancements. In particular, these conventions might incorporate lessening sodium consumption, keeping away from handled food varieties and liquor, devouring all the more new products of the soil, expanding actual work, and taking enhancements like omega-3 unsaturated fats, probiotics, and cancer prevention agents.

Try not to smoke and drink liquor, as this can harm the kidneys and liver.

It is likewise essential to accept the drug as endorsed by your primary care physician and circle back to customary lab tests to screen kidney and liver capability. At last, look for clinical exhortation from a certified medical services supplier before starting any therapy program.

A. Day 1-7: Detoxification

Day 1: Begin your detoxification by drinking a lot of liquids. Water is the most ideal decision and you ought to intend to polish off somewhere around 8 glasses every day. You can likewise incorporate homegrown teas and newly squeezed leafy foods juices. What's more, it is prescribed to supplant your customary dinners with feasts that are low in fat, sugar, and salt. This will assist with flushing out poisons from your body.

Day 2: On day two, you ought to begin to integrate food sources that are wealthy in fiber into your eating regimen. This can incorporate entire grains, organic products, vegetables, and vegetables. Eating these food sources will assist with purifying your stomach-related framework and work on the well-being of your kidneys and liver.

Day 3: Integrate all the more new foods grown from the ground into your eating routine. These are loaded with fundamental nutrients and minerals that can assist with detoxifying your body and work on your general well-being. You can likewise include lean proteins like lean meats, fish, and egg whites.

Day 4: Spotlight on eating protein-rich food varieties like nuts, seeds, and vegetables. These food varieties are loaded with fundamental amino acids that can assist with supporting sound liver and kidney capabilities. You ought to likewise incorporate food sources that are high in cancer prevention agents like berries and dim mixed greens.

Day 5: Consolidate food varieties that are high in omega-3 unsaturated fats into your eating regimen. These unsaturated fats are fundamental for keeping up with solid liver and kidney capabilities. Great wellsprings of omega-3 unsaturated fats incorporate fish, pecans, flaxseed, and chia seeds.

Day 6: Drink a lot of liquids and ensure that you are getting sufficient rest. This will assist with flushing out poisons from your body and keep up with sound liver and kidney capabilities.

Day 7: On the last day of your detoxification, you ought to zero in on devouring food varieties that are high in probiotics. Probiotics are advantageous microbes that can assist with working on your absorption and backing sound liver and kidney capabilities. Great wellsprings of probiotics incorporate yogurt, sauerkraut, and kimchi.

B. Day 8-10: Stimulating the Kidneys and Liver

Eight: Invigorating the kidney and liver should be possible through dietary and way-of-life changes. Eating a fair eating routine of leafy foods, entire grains, and incline protein can assist with supporting legitimate kidney and liver capability. Likewise, drinking a lot of water every day and keeping away from unreasonable liquor admission can assist with keeping these crucial organs sound.

Nine: Customary activity is likewise a significant piece of invigorating the kidney and liver. The practice assists with expanding dissemination to these organs, which can assist them with working all the more productively. Furthermore, captivating exercises, for example, yoga and reflection can assist with decreasing pressure, which can likewise assist with supporting the soundness of the kidneys and liver.

Ten: Enhancements may likewise help animate the kidney and liver. Certain nutrients and minerals, like vitamin B6, magnesium, and zinc can assist with supporting the organs' well-being and capability. Natural cures, for example, dandelion root and milk thorn, may likewise be useful in reinforcing kidney and liver capability.

C. Days 11-14: Liver Cleansing Diet

Day 11

Breakfast: New natural product smoothie with banana, berries, and almond milk

Nibble: Detoxifying green tea and apples

Lunch: Vegetable soup with grain, lentils, and different vegetables

Nibble: Blended nuts and seeds

Supper: Barbecued salmon with earthy-colored rice and steamed vegetables

Day 12

Breakfast: Detoxifying green smoothie with spinach, banana, and almond milk

Nibble: Celery sticks with hummus

Lunch: Quinoa salad with vegetables and a lemon vinaigrette

Nibble: Carrot and cucumber sticks with tahini plunge

Supper: Prepared yam with steamed broccoli and a side of steamed greens

Day 13

Breakfast: Oats with berries and almond milk

Nibble: Detoxifying green tea and apples

Lunch: Vegetable pan-fried food with earthy-colored rice

Nibble: Celery sticks with nut margarine

Supper: Barbecued chicken with yam wedges and a side of steamed greens

Day 14

Breakfast: Detoxifying green smoothie with spinach, and banana.

D. Days 15-19: Kidney Cleansing

Day 15

Breakfast: Green smoothie made with kale, spinach, cucumber, celery, and lemon juice.

Nibble: Celery sticks with almond spread.

Lunch: Quinoa salad with kidney beans, ringer peppers, tomatoes, and a lemon vinaigrette.

Nibble: Apple cuts with pecans.

Supper: Heated salmon with simmered asparagus and a side of earthy-colored rice.

Day 16

Breakfast: Cereal with blueberries and almonds.

Nibble: Carrot sticks with hummus.

Lunch: Lentil soup with a side of steamed broccoli.

Nibble: Celery sticks with almond margarine.

Supper: Prepared salmon with cooked Brussels sprouts and a side of quinoa.

Day 17

Breakfast: Greek yogurt with berries and granola.

Nibble: Apple cuts with pecans.

Lunch: Chickpea and vegetable pan-fried food with earthy-colored rice.

Nibble: Celery sticks with hummus.

Supper: Prepared cod with cooked cauliflower and a side of quinoa.

Day 18

Breakfast: Green smoothie made with kale, spinach, cucumber, celery, and lemon juice.

Nibble: Carrot sticks with almond margarine.

Lunch: Kale salad with kidney beans, chime peppers, tomatoes, and a lemon vinaigrette.

Nibble: Apple cuts with pecans.

Supper: Prepared tilapia with broiled asparagus and a side of earthy-colored rice.

Day 19

Breakfast: Oats with blueberries and almonds.

Nibble: Celery sticks with hummus.

Lunch: Lentil soup with a side of steamed broccoli.

Nibble: Carrot sticks with almond margarine.

Supper: Prepared cod with cooked Brussels sprouts and a side of quinoa.

Chapter 6: Post-cure care for Kidney and Fatty Liver Cure

Post-cure care is a critical aspect of recovery for individuals who have undergone treatment for kidney and fatty liver disease. After treatment, it is important to maintain a healthy lifestyle and follow specific guidelines to prevent the recurrence of these conditions.

For individuals who have undergone treatment for kidney disease, post-cure care involves managing blood pressure, monitoring fluid intake, and maintaining a healthy diet. It is important to limit the intake of sodium, potassium, and phosphorus and increase the consumption of fresh fruits and vegetables. Regular exercise and staying hydrated can also aid in the recovery process.

For individuals who have undergone treatment for fatty liver disease, post-cure care involves maintaining a healthy weight, following a balanced diet, and staying physically active. It is important to limit the intake of saturated and trans fats and increase the consumption of fruits, vegetables, and whole grains. Avoiding alcohol and other harmful substances can also improve liver health.

In both cases, regular check-ups with a healthcare professional and following any medication regimens prescribed are critical for long-term management and prevention of complications. With proper post-cure care, individuals can successfully recover from kidney and fatty liver disease and maintain a healthy lifestyle.

Post-cure care for kidney disease:

Follow a healthy diet: After receiving treatment for kidney disease, it is essential to follow a healthy and balanced diet. One should limit the intake of salt, potassium, and phosphorus. Foods high in potassium include bananas, avocados, oranges, and tomatoes. Foods high in phosphorus include dairy products, nuts, and beans. A dietician or a healthcare provider can provide more information on what foods to eat or avoid.

Stay hydrated: Drinking plenty of water helps to keep the kidneys functioning correctly. One should drink at least eight glasses of water per day, and more if advised by a healthcare provider.

Monitor blood pressure: High blood pressure can damage the kidneys. One should monitor their blood pressure regularly and take medication as prescribed by a healthcare provider.

Exercise regularly: Regular exercise can help to keep the kidneys healthy. One should aim for at least 30 minutes of exercise per day, such as brisk walking, jogging, or swimming.

Avoid smoking and alcohol: Smoking and alcohol can damage the kidneys and worsen kidney disease. One should avoid smoking and limit alcohol intake or avoid it entirely.

Post-cure care for fatty liver disease:

Maintain a healthy weight: Being overweight or obese is a significant risk factor for fatty liver disease. One should aim to maintain a healthy weight by following a healthy diet and regular exercise.

Avoid alcohol: Alcohol is a significant cause of fatty liver disease. One should avoid alcohol or limit it to a maximum of one drink per day for women and two drinks per day for men.

Control diabetes: Diabetes is a risk factor for fatty liver disease. One should aim to control their blood sugar levels by following a healthy diet, taking medication as prescribed, and monitoring blood sugar levels regularly.

Avoid certain medications: Some medications can cause or worsen fatty liver disease. One should avoid taking medications without consulting a healthcare provider.

Get vaccinated: Hepatitis A and B can cause liver damage and worsen fatty liver disease. One should get vaccinated against hepatitis A and B.

Post-cure care is an essential aspect of the treatment process for kidney and fatty liver disease. Following a healthy diet, staying hydrated, monitoring blood pressure, exercising regularly, avoiding smoking and alcohol, maintaining a healthy weight, controlling diabetes, avoiding certain medications, and getting vaccinated can help to prevent the recurrence or worsening of these conditions. It is essential to consult a healthcare provider for more information on post-cure care measures specific to individual needs.

Conclusion

The kidney and liver fix is a characteristic, all-encompassing way to deal with assisting the body with recuperating itself and keep up with ideal well-being. It consolidates dietary changes, supplementation, and way-of-life changes to assist with managing the body's normal purifying cycles and help the body detoxify and revive. Generally speaking, the kidney and liver fix is a protected and successful way to deal with further developing well-being, forestalling sickness, and reestablishing harmony and imperativeness. Albeit further exploration is expected to completely comprehend the advantages of this methodology, the accessible proof recommends that it tends to be a successful method for working on general well-being and prosperity.

Accordingly, the kidney and liver fix is a compelling and safe approach to further developing well-being and forestalling infection. It is essential to recollect that weight control plans, supplementation, and way-of-life changes ought to be custom fitted to the person, as every individual's body is extraordinary. At long last, it is suggested that people look for direction from medical care proficient to guarantee that the kidney and liver fix is carried out in a protected and viable way.

If you enjoyed reading this book, please give this book a favorable review. Thanks

Printed in France by Amazon
Brétigny-sur-Orge, FR

16156254R00060